Andrés Martínez Esteve
Francisco Javier García Gómez

Primary Adrenal Lymphoma and Nuclear Medicine

Andrés Martínez Esteve
Francisco Javier García Gómez

Primary Adrenal Lymphoma and Nuclear Medicine

LAP LAMBERT Academic Publishing

Impressum / Imprint

Bibliografische Information der Deutschen Nationalbibliothek: Die Deutsche Nationalbibliothek verzeichnet diese Publikation in der Deutschen Nationalbibliografie; detaillierte bibliografische Daten sind im Internet über http://dnb.d-nb.de abrufbar.

Alle in diesem Buch genannten Marken und Produktnamen unterliegen warenzeichen-, marken- oder patentrechtlichem Schutz bzw. sind Warenzeichen oder eingetragene Warenzeichen der jeweiligen Inhaber. Die Wiedergabe von Marken, Produktnamen, Gebrauchsnamen, Handelsnamen, Warenbezeichnungen u.s.w. in diesem Werk berechtigt auch ohne besondere Kennzeichnung nicht zu der Annahme, dass solche Namen im Sinne der Warenzeichen- und Markenschutzgesetzgebung als frei zu betrachten wären und daher von jedermann benutzt werden dürften.

Bibliographic information published by the Deutsche Nationalbibliothek: The Deutsche Nationalbibliothek lists this publication in the Deutsche Nationalbibliografie; detailed bibliographic data are available in the Internet at http://dnb.d-nb.de.

Any brand names and product names mentioned in this book are subject to trademark, brand or patent protection and are trademarks or registered trademarks of their respective holders. The use of brand names, product names, common names, trade names, product descriptions etc. even without a particular marking in this work is in no way to be construed to mean that such names may be regarded as unrestricted in respect of trademark and brand protection legislation and could thus be used by anyone.

Coverbild / Cover image: www.ingimage.com

Verlag / Publisher:
LAP LAMBERT Academic Publishing
ist ein Imprint der / is a trademark of
OmniScriptum GmbH & Co. KG
Bahnhofstraße 28, 66111 Saarbrücken, Deutschland / Germany
Email: info@omniscriptum.com

Herstellung: siehe letzte Seite /
Printed at: see last page
ISBN: 978-3-659-79064-5

Table of contents

The term lymphoma includes a heterogeneous group of malignancies arising from lymphoid tissue, with varied clinical and biological features. Currently, the estimated incidence for Hodgkin and Non-Hodgkin lymphomas reached up to 2.5 and 11.7 age standardised rate per 100,000 respectively. This makes the lymphoma become a major public health problem in most industrialized countries.

Regarding primary adrenal lymphoma is an extremely rare entity accounting for less than 1% of all non-Hodgkin's lymphoma cases and 3% of extranodal lymphoma.

With this book, we aim to reflect a detailed review of reported medical literature and focusing on the diagnostic aspects.

In the first chapter, we will concisely explain the key points of the entity as to their generalities, histological types, therapeutic possibilities, etc. intending to lead the reader to grasp the root of the diagnostic problem.

Second chapter is intended as discussion focusing on the Positron Emission Tomography/Computed Tomography (PET/CT) role. This hybrid imaging technique has been established in the last decade and has changed the traditional paradigm, leading major changes in the diagnosis and management of these patients.

A detailed review of the *state of the art of* 18F-FDG PET/CT in the initial staging, evaluation of bone marrow involvement, assessment of the early and final response to treatment, as well as in the routine follow-up of lymphoma could be found in this chapter.

Finally, in the last chapter we touched on the specificities of primary adrenal lymphoma. According to the imagenological nature of the book, a historical review of the very few published papers is done, from the oldest techniques to the PET/CT role in the present context.

The highly focus on practice in this manual is intended to serve as an useful learning tool for medical students, junior doctors and specialists in different areas and, of course, for residents and specialists in nuclear medicine. For this reason, and because we know you'll really appreciate having high quality images in this book, we have provided our group images which will be available at the following QR code:

Andrés Martínez Esteve

Francisco Javier García Gómez

Chapter 1.

Overview of Lymphoma

Introduction

The term lymphoma includes a heterogeneous group of malignancies arising from lymphoid tissue, with varied clinical and biological features. It is characterized by the formation of solid tumors in the immune system [1].

Currently, the estimated incidence in Europe for Hodgkin and Non-Hodgkin`s lymphomas reached up to 2.5 and 11.7 age standardised rate per 100,000 people respectively [2, 3]. On the other hand, it is estimate that there are nearly 20 cases of Non-Hodgkin's lymphoma for every 100,000 people and around three cases in every 100,000 people in the United States of America [4, 5].
This makes the lymphoma become a major public health problem in most industrialized countries.

The classification of the malignant lymphomas has undergone significant reappraisal over the past five decades, resulted from insights gained through the application of immunologic and molecular techniques, as well a better understanding of the clinical aspects of lymphoma through advances in diagnosis, staging, and treatment [6].

Currently, the World Health Organization (WHO) classification of neoplasms of the hematopoietic and lymphoid tissues, updated in 2008, represents a worldwide consensus on the diagnosis of these tumors, adopted for use by pathologists, clinicians, and basic scientists [7].

WHO classification of tumors of hematopoietic and lymphoid tissues is detailed explain in Table 1.

Because of the imagenologic nature of this book, we will concisely explain the key points of the most common types (Hodgkin and Non-Hodgkin's lymphomas) as to their generalities, histological types, therapeutic possibilities, etc. intending to lead the reader to grasp the root of the diagnostic problem.

Mature B-cell neoplasms

Chronic lymphocytic leukemia/small lymphocytic lymphoma

B-cell prolymphocytic leukemia

Splenic marginal zone lymphoma

Hairy cell leukemia

Splenic lymphoma/leukemia, unclassifiable[*]

    Splenic diffuse red pulp small B-cell lymphoma[*]

    Hairy cell leukemia variant[*]

Lymphoplasmacytic lymphoma

    Waldenström macroglobulinemia

Heavy chain diseases

    α Heavy chain disease

    γ Heavy chain disease

    μ Heavy chain disease

Plasma cell myeloma

Solitary plasmacytoma of bone

Extraosseous plasmacytoma

Extranodal marginal zone lymphoma of mucosa-associated lymphoid tissue (MALT lymphoma)

N dal marginal zone lymphoma

    Pediatric nodal marginal zone lymphoma[*]

Follicular lymphoma

    Pediatric follicular lymphoma[*]

Primary cutaneous follicle centre lymphoma

Mantle cell lymphoma

Diffuse large B-cell lymphoma (DLBCL), NOS

    T-cell/histiocyte rich large B-cell lymphoma

Primary DLBCL of the CNS

Primary cutaneous DLBCL, leg type

EBV-positive DLBCL of the elderly[*]

DLBCL associated with chronic inflammation

Lymphomatoid granulomatosis

Primary mediastinal (thymic) large B-cell lymphoma

Intravascular large B-cell lymphoma

ALK-positive large B-cell lymphoma

Plasmablastic lymphoma

Large B-cell lymphoma arising in HHV8-associated multicentric Castleman disease

Primary effusion lymphoma

Burkitt lymphoma

B-cell lymphoma, unclassifiable, with features intermediate between diffuse large B-cell lymphoma and Burkitt lymphoma

B-cell lymphoma, unclassifiable, with features intermediate between diffuse large B-cell lymphoma and classical Hodgkin lymphoma

Mature T-cell and NK-cell neoplasms

T-cell prolymphocytic leukemia

T-cell large granular lymphocytic leukemia

Chronic lymphoproliferative disorder of NK cells[*]

Aggressive NK-cell leukemia

Systemic EBV-positive T-cell lymphoproliferative disease of childhood

Hydroa vacciniforme-like lymphoma

Adult T-cell leukemia/lymphoma

Extranodal NK/T-cell lymphoma, nasal type

Enteropathy-associated T-cell lymphoma

Hepatosplenic T-cell lymphoma

Subcutaneous panniculitis-like T-cell lymphoma

Mycosis fungoides

Sézary syndrome

Primary cutaneous CD30$^+$ T-cell lymphoproliferative disorders

    Lymphomatoid papulosis

    Primary cutaneous anaplastic large cell lymphoma

Primary cutaneous γδ T-cell lymphoma

Primary cutaneous CD8$^+$ aggressive epidermotropic cytotoxic T-cell lymphoma[*]

Primary cutaneous CD4$^+$ small/medium T-cell lymphoma[*]

Peripheral T-cell lymphoma, NOS

Angioimmunoblastic T-cell lymphoma

Anaplastic large cell lymphoma, ALK-positive

Anaplastic large cell lymphoma, ALK-negative[*]

Hodgkin lymphoma

Nodular lymphocyte predominant Hodgkin lymphoma

Classical Hodgkin lymphoma

Nodular sclerosis classical Hodgkin lymphoma

Lymphocyte-rich classical Hodgkin lymphoma

Mixed cellularity classical Hodgkin lymphoma

Lymphocyte-depleted classical Hodgkin lymphoma

Histiocytic and dendritic cell neoplasms
Histiocytic sarcoma Langerhans cell histiocytosis Langerhans cell sarcoma Interdigitating dendritic cell sarcoma Follicular dendritic cell sarcoma Fibroblastic reticular cell tumor Intermediate dendritic cell tumor Disseminated juvenile xanthogranuloma
Posttransplantation lymphoproliferative disorders (PTLDs)

Early lesions
 	
    Plasmacytic hyperplasia
 	
    Infectious mononucleosis–like PTLD
 	
Polymorphic PTLD
 	
Monomorphic PTLD (B- and T/NK-cell types)[†]
 	
Classical Hodgkin lymphoma type PTLD[†]

Table 1: 2008 updated WHO classification of tumors of hematopoietic and lymphoid. Adapted from [8]: Campo E, Swerdlow SH, Harris NL, et al. The 2008 WHO classification of lymphoid neoplasms and beyond: evolving concepts and practical applications. Blood. 2011;117:5019-5032.

NOS indicates not otherwise specified; ALK, anaplastic lymphoma kinase; HHV8, human herpesvirus 8; and NK, natural killer. * These histologic types are provisional entities for which the WHO Working Group felt there was insufficient evidence to recognize as distinct diseases at this time. [†] These lesions are classified according to the leukemia or lymphoma to which they correspond.

Hodgkin's lymphoma:

Hodgkin's lymphoma is a B cell–derived cancer, being one of the most common lymphomas. In this entity, the tumor cells are known as Reed-Sternberg cells and are usually very rare in the tissue. This lymphoid malignancy involves peripheral lymphatic nodes but it is also not uncommon that can affect non-lymphatic organs such as liver, lung, and bone marrow. This entity can occur at any age but is most prevalent between the ages of 15 and 40 and after the age of 55, according to the American Cancer Society.

The most common form of progression occurs as lymphatic dissemination to nearby lymph areas, being a characteristic pattern of progression this disease. It can also occur by vicinity and hematogenous spread.

Most patients are diagnosed upon detection of cervical and mediastinal lymph nodes. Up to 40% of patients suffer fever, night sweats, and weight loss consistent with constitutional or "B-symptoms" [9]. In about 40% of classical Hodgkin's lymphoma in the Western world, as well as in more than 90% of pediatric cases of Hodgkin's lymphoma in Central America, Reed-Sternberg cells are latently infected by Ebstein-Barr Virus [10].

Regarding its initial stating, 18F-FDG PET/CT has become an essential tool. Its role in the early diagnosis, as well as the Ann Arbor classification, the Deauville criteria for interim PET and monitoring in Hodgkin's lymphoma will be widely developed in chapter 2.

Respect to the treatment of these patients, is based on radiotherapy regimens (usually from 32 to 40 Gy) and chemotherapy mainly with ADVB (Adriamicine, Bleomicine, Vinblastine, Dacarbacepine) scheme depending on stage and clinical risk factors. After introduction of multi-agent chemotherapy and improved radiation techniques, the prognosis of Hodgkin's lymphoma has substantially improved. Up to 90% of patients can be rendered disease-free after five years [11].

Non-Hodgkin's lymphoma

As well as Hodgkin's lymphoma, Non-Hodgkin's lymphomas are a heterogeneous group of malignancies of the lymphoid system. However, is much less predictable than Hodgkin lymphoma and has a far greater predilection to disseminate to extranodal sites [12].

This entity has been classified as B-cell and T-cell neoplasms. In this vein, B-cell lymphomas account for approximately 90% of all lymphomas, being follicular lymphoma and diffuse large B-cell lymphoma the 2 most common histological disease entities [13].

As for his clinic, it is quite similar to Hodgkin's lymphoma related, with subtle differences in the clinical manifestations. In this sense, extralymphatic spread, mesenteric lymphatic involvement, liver infiltration without splenic involvement, infiltration of bone marrow or leukemic expression are most common than in Hodgkin's lymphoma.

The Ann Arbor Staging Classification is used routinely to classify the extent of disease, and the International Prognostic Index has been used to define prognostic subgroups [13].

As in the case of Hodgkin's lymphoma, the utility of PET/CT in all stages of diagnosis and monitoring are largely detailed in chapter 2.

Treatment of Non-Hodgkin's lymphoma depends on the histologic type and stage. In asymptomatic patients with indolent forms of advanced Non-Hodgkin's lymphoma, treatment may be deferred until the patient becomes symptomatic as the disease progresses. Regarding treatment options for aggressive, noncontiguous Stage II/III/IV Adult Non-Hodgkin's lymphoma, several studies established R-CHOP as the standard regimen for newly diagnosed patients. The majority of patients who receive radiation are usually treated on only one side of the diaphragm with dose of radiation that usually varies from 25 Gy to 50 Gy.

Primary lymphoma

Primary lymphoma is referred to those lymphomas which mainly involves the extranodal tissue. There are several reports of primary lymphoma in the literature, being the central nervous system (CNS), gastrointestinal (GI) tract and other endocrine organs (such as adrenal glands or thyroid gland) the most frequently affected [14]. There are also other reports were involvement of other tissues as the urinary bladder, or bone is provided [15-17].

The Primary Adrenal lymphoma will be explained in detail in the Chapter 3.

Primary CNS lymphoma

Primary CNS lymphoma is a rare entity which is limited to the brain, eyes, meninges, cranial nerves and spinal cord, without systemic disease. The primary CNS lymphoma comprising 2.2% of all tumors [18] in this location, most of them (95%) are aggressive diffuse large B-cell lymphomas. Although most are sporadic, is fairly common in HIV-infected patient or other immunosuppressed state as corticosteroid therapy following organ transplantation [19].

The diagnosis of primary CNS lymphoma is done mostly by stereotactic biopsy or by flow cytometric analysis of cerebrospinal fluid lymphocytes [20]. Magnetic resonance imaging is the main tool in the detection and monitoring of this disease. Nevertheless, findings in this technique are usually non-specific, and besides, differentiation from other diseases such as metastases, glioblastoma or demyelinating dementia may be difficult [21]. Whole-body 18F-FDG PET/CT has an important role in staging and exclusion of systemic involvement. Usually, primary CNS lymphoma show homogeneous and high avidity 18F-FDG uptake [22]. The role of Rituximab is unclear because its low CNS penetration.

For treatment, due to the rarity of this entity, there is no treatment algorithm established. In this context, high-dose methotrexate-based chemotherapy is currently considered the standard of care as induction therapy [20]. For consolidation of treatment, whole-body radiotherapy has been proposed, however, neurotoxicity is a very important limitation when applying it [23]. Furthermore, high-dose chemotherapy and autologous stem cell transplantation have been proposed in relapsed/refractory primary CNS lymphoma and as a consolidation therapy.

Poor prognostic factors include: age older than 50 years, performance status >1, elevated LDH serum level, elevated cerebrospinal fluid protein concentration, involvement of nonhemispheric areas of the brain.

Primary GI tract lymphoma

Lymphomas of the GI tract are the most common type of primary extranodal lymphomas, accounting for 5 to 10% of all non-Hodgkin's lymphoma, varying according to the geographical zones [24, 25]. Most primary GI tract lymphomas arise in the stomach. At presentation, patients are usually asymptomatic, but abdominal pain, intestinal obstruction, and diarrhea may occur [26].

Endosonography, radiological examination and 18F-FDG PET/CT are used in the detection of this entity.

Rituximab has shown efficacy treating B cell lymphomas becoming an optimal therapeutic modality for localized primary GI tract diffuse large B-cell lymphomas. However, patients unfit for Rituximab treatment, radical surgery may be considered as a therapeutic modality [27].

Primary thyroid lymphoma

Primary thyroid lymphoma is a rare disease comprising 1 to 5% of all thyroid malignancies [28]. As in other primary lymphomas, B-cell is the most common origin, being diffuse large B-cell lymphoma and low-grade B-cell lymphoma of mucosa-associated lymphoid tissue (MALT) the most common histological subtypes [29].

Treatment depends on histological subtype, and for aggressive diffuse large B-cell lymphoma it is based on chemotherapy (CHOP), adding radiotherapy in cases of localized aggressive lymphoma [30].

Primary lymphoma of the urinary bladder

Primary lymphoma of the urinary bladder are extremely rare accounting for <1% of all bladder tumors and 0.2% of all extranodal lymphomas [31]. Most of them are low-grade lymphomas, being the B-cell derived non-Hodgkin's lymphomas of the MALT type the common subtype. On the other hand, high-grade lymphomas are rare comprising up to 20% of cases [32]. The most common symptoms are haematuria, urinary frequency, dysuria and nocturia [33].

In the diagnosis of this pathology, ultrasound and subsequent cystoscopy is usually the initial investigation. Bone marrow biopsy and 18F-FDG PET/CT are commonly used in a high-grade tumor, because the possibility of systemic involvement increases [32, 33].

The treatment of choice is a combination of chemotherapy (CHOP regimen) and radiotherapy. Radiotherapy alone may be used in tumors of low-grade type and small size [33].

Primary bone lymphoma

Primary lymphoma of the bone comprises approximately 3% of all primary malignant tumors and 1% of all lymphomas [34]. Primary bone lymphoma arises from the medullary cavity. The most commonly sites of involvement in this pathology are the extremities [35]. As with other primary lymphomas, the most common subtype is lymphoma of B-cell origin [36]. At presentation, patients usually present pain, swelling, pathologic fractures.

For diagnosis, conventional radiography, scintigraphic studies (bone scintigraphy) which alters the prognosis and treatment if it detects multifocal involvement, CT, MRI and 18F-FDG PET/CT, which a currently study has suggested that it is a sensitive imaging modality for diagnosis and treatment response evaluation [34, 37].

For treatment, combination of chemotherapy and radiotherapy is superior to radiotherapy alone, which has a poor five-year overall survival rate [38, 39].

Chapter 2.

PET/CT in lymphoma

Introduction

Currently, the management of patients with history of lymphoma in everyday clinical practice is determined by histology, initial staging, tumor size and involvement of individual organs, being necessary to delimit between patients who will be treated by chemotherapy of those who could benefit from radiotherapy. The most important factors influencing physician decisions and prognosis are histologic subtype and extent of disease. In this sense, Ann Arbor classification was introduced in 1971 and being still in use [40]. In the Initial Staging subsection the Ann Arbor classification will be explained in detail.

For decades, both initial staging and evaluation of treatment response in patients with lymphoma were based on morphological CT images and bone marrow biopsy. On the one hand, contrast enhanced CT has related a high sensitivity for detecting lymph node and visceral involvement with morphological changes, while on the other allows detecting infiltration of bone marrow which conditions the therapeutic strategy and prognosis. However, these techniques are not exempt from limitations, due to the difficulty in determining the presence or absence of nodal and extranodal disease without morphologic changes, which can lead to equivocal findings. On the other hand, bone marrow biopsy may not be representative in case of limited involvement [41-43]. As expected, incorrect initial staging and assessment of response to treatment will have important consequences for the patient.

The incursion of the Positron Emission Tomography/Computed Tomography (PET/CT) in the last decade has changed this paradigm, leading major changes in the diagnosis and management of these patients, allowing the study of the whole-body while assessing morphological and metabolic changes through a minimally invasive technique. PET/CT also allows a quantitative assessment of the degree of cell activity, which is essential to determine the degree of malignancy of the lesions and quantitatively assess the response to treatment.

The information provided by this technique improves the initial staging, prognostic approach and choice a proper treatment plan, assess the response to therapy and monitoring for diagnosis of recurrence and restaging of lymphoma [44-45].

Thus, it has become a powerful tool for nodal and extranodal evaluation in patients with lymphoma.

A report by the National Comprehensive Cancer Network (NCCN) in 2007 mentioned that PET/CT with 2-deoxy-2-[18F]-fluoro-D-glucose (18F-FDG) for assessment of lymphomas could reach more than 50% of the total PET scans [46]. Today it has been exceeded in any PET reference center.

18F-FDG radiotracer allows evaluating lymphoproliferative disease by imaging and quantitating the glycolytic metabolism within the tumor cells. Thereby, PET/CT with 18F-FDG is a noninvasive, semiquantitative whole-body imaging technique that can detect malignancies through both anatomical and functional approaches.

Nevertheless, at this point it should be remembered that 18F-FDG is not a specific tracer for tumor tissue, and it will also be retained in high glucose metabolism processes, such as inflammation, infection, etc.

Each histologic subtypes of lymphoma differ in molecular characteristics and biologic behavior so 18F-FDG avidity will be variable due to the different degrees of malignancy and proliferative activity.

Most lymphoma subtypes have been shown highly avidity for 18F-FDG, especially in aggressive lymphomas with a higher rate of cell proliferation. These include Hodgkin disease, diffuse large B-cell lymphoma, mantle cell lymphoma, Burkitt lymphoma, lymphoblastic lymphoma, anaplastic large T-cell lymphoma, angioimmunoblastic T-cell lymphoma, and natural killer/T-cell lymphoma, with avidity rates near than 100%. Metabolic and morphologic information provided by PET/CT becomes the most sensitive and specific imaging test in patients with these histologic subtypes [47].

On the contrary, lower 18F-FDG avidity has been reported for indolent lymphoma subtypes such as small lymphocytic lymphoma, peripheral T-cell lymphoma, anaplastic large T-cell lymphoma and extranodal marginal zone lymphomas, including the mucosa-associated lymphoid tissue (MALT), marginal zone lymphoma and splenic marginal zone lymphoma [48-50]. Different 18F-FDG avidities are given in Table 2.

Histologic subtype	18F-FDG avidity
Hodgkin disease:	
Classical Hodgkin's lymphoma	High
Nodular sclerosis	Moderate – High
Aggressive Non-Hodgkin lymphoma:	
Diffuse large B cell lymphoma	Moderate – High
Burkitt lymphoma	High
Peripheral T cell lymphoma	Low – High
Anaplastic large cell lymphoma	High
Mantle cell lymphoma	Moderate
Indolent Non-Hodgkin lymphoma:	
Follicular lymphoma	Low – High
Lymphoplasmacytic lymphoma	Low – Moderate
Nodal marginal zone lymphoma	Null – High
Extranodal marginal zone lymphoma	Null – High
Small lymphocytic lymphoma	Null – High
Cutaneous T cell lymphoma	Null - Moderate

Table 2. 18F-FDG avidities, modified from [50].

Despite this, individual characteristics will condition the degree of 18F-FDG uptake.

This data is clinically important, as it is known that there is a direct correlation between the degree of malignancy and 18F-FDG uptake, resulting in lower diagnostic yield of PET in the indolent or low-grade lymphomas [51].

17

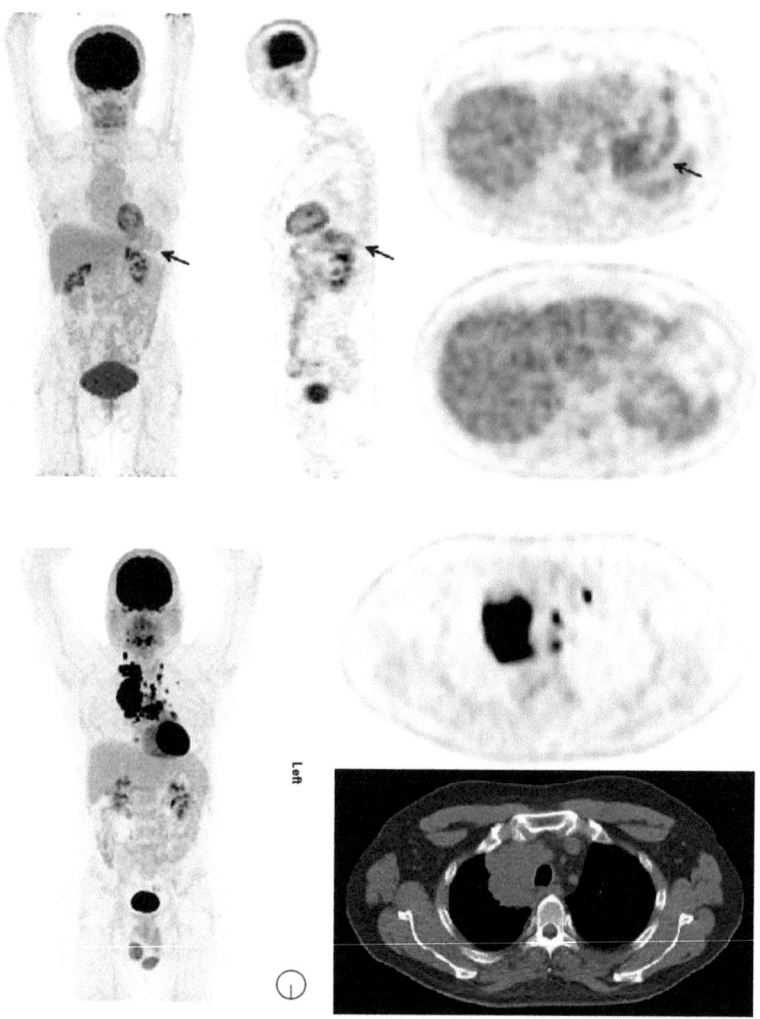

Figure 1: Patients with different 18F-FDG avidities at initial staging PET/CT scans. Below patient showed slight increased radiotracer uptake in the gastric fundus (arrows) reaching a SUVmax of 4.3, corresponding with MALT lymphoma. Above patient characterized by predominantly mediastinal nodal involvement, regarding a high rate of cell proliferation with SUVmax of 35.1 in the context of Nodular Sclerosis Hodgkin's Lymphoma stage II.

However, the optimal application of 18F-FDG PET/CT scans in lymphoma remains problematic because of several variables, as well as the meaning of a positive PET by the absence of clear standards for PET/CT interpretation [47].

Recently, the recommendations were upgraded in an attempt to normalize the international clinical practice regarding evaluation, staging, and response assessment formally including PET/CT into the standard staging and response assessment of 18F-FDG-avid lymphomas [52]. Below we will detail the implications of PET in each of these milestones in patients with lymphoma.

As a general guideline, basic recommendations for proper acquisition of 18F-FDG PET/CT scans in patients with lymphoma will be explained in Table 3.

Other non-18F-FDG radiotracers have also proved useful in the evaluation of lymphoma in preclinical studies. Thus, the 18F-FLT (3'-[18F]fluoro-3'-deoxythymidine) behaves as a cell proliferation marker which has demonstrated good results in predicting disease-free survival. 18F-FLT has also has demonstrated its superiority in differentiating between viable tumor and inflammatory changes leading improving the specificity of the study [53-56].

In the other hand, Fludarabine is a drug used in the treatment of indolent lymphoma, that has also been labeled with 18F, showing its utility in lymphomas in which the role of 18F-FDG is more limited [57].

Parameter	Recommendations
Patient preparation	Fast of at least 6 hours. No active exercise before to the scan acquisition. Consider sedation in case of inability to maintain posture during the study.
Blood glucose level	Lower than 180 mg/dL.
18F-FDG dose	3.7-7.4 MBq/kg (0.1-0.2 mCi/kg) body weight, minimum 185 MBq. Proper hydration post-injection. Administration of a diuretic (10–20 mg i.v. furosemide).
PET acquisition	60 minutes post-injection of 18F-FDG. If delay scan: 180 minutes post-injection.
Images reconstruction	Iterative reconstruction: 4 iterations and 8 subsets. If TRUETOF reconstruction available: 2 iterations and 21 subsets.
Timing of scan	Pretreatment scans are mandatory. Post-treatment scans at least 6-8 weeks after chemo(immuno)therapy or 8-12 weeks after radiotherapy.

Table 3: Recommendations for PET acquisition. Modified from [47].

PET/CT at initial staging

The initial staging of the disease define the location, extent of the disease and suggests prognostic information. Furthermore, allows comparison with other studies, and provides a baseline image as a reference for assessing response [58]. In this moment, PET/CT is already widely used for pretreatment staging, also being widely introduced in the assessment of the response. Although clinical examination is still important, baseline PET/CT is critical to increase the effectiveness of the assessment of the response of the treatment [59].

The latest established consensus is that PET/CT should be recommended for routine staging of 18F-FDG avid nodal lymphomas (all histologies except chronic lymphocytic leukemia / small lymphocytic lymphoma, lymphoplasmacytic lymphoma / Waldenström's macroglobulinemia, mycosis fungoides, and marginal zone Non-Hodgkin lymphomas, unless there is a suspicion of aggressive transformation) as the gold standard [60].

In the patient staged with 18F-FDG PET/CT, every nodal or extranodal radiotracer uptake which cannot be justified by any physiological increased uptake, must be considered as lymphomatous involvement, including spleen, liver, bone, thyroid, and so on. A measurable lymphadenopathy should have a longest diameter of at least 1.5 cm. Regarding extranodal level, a measurable lesion should be at least 1 cm in the longest diameter. Thirdly, a nodal mass of 10 cm or greater than a third of the transthoracic diameter is defined as bulky mass [52].

Concerning splenic involvement, it is best determined by 18F-FDG PET/CT and may be characterized by homogeneous splenomegaly, diffuse infiltration with miliary lesions, focal nodular lesions, or a large solitary mass [61].

Cheson group recommends a modified Ann Arbor classification for accurate anatomic description of disease extent. However, in clinical practice tends to treat patients according to prognostic and risk factors. This implies a practical division in limited (stages I and II, non-bulky) or advanced (stages III or IV) disease. Stage II bulky disease is considered as

21

limited or advanced disease, depending on histology and a number of prognostic factors. The designation E for extranodal disease is relevant only for limited extranodal disease in the absence of nodal involvement (IE) or in patients with stage II disease and direct extension to a non-nodal site. Secondly, suffixes A and B, according to the absence (A) or presence (B) of disease-related symptoms (known as "Symptoms B"), are only required for Hodgkin lymphoma [52].

As for the primary extranodal disease, different recommendations have been published and must to be considered depending on the histological type and/or extent of the disease [62-63].

Table 4 shows the Ann Arbor classification modified by Cheson et al which is in force.

Below you could find some specific aspects for each histologic subtype, divided into Hodgkin's lymphoma, and aggressive or indolent Non-Hodgkin lymphoma.

Stage	Involvement	Extranodal status
Limited		
I	One node or a group of adjacent nodes.	Single extranodal lesion without nodal involvement.
II	Two or more nodal groups on the same side of diaphragm.	Stage I or II by nodal extent with limited adjacent extranodal involvement.
II bulky	Stage II with bulky mass.	Not applicable.
Advanced		
III	Nodal involvement on both sides of the diaphragm, or supradiaphragmatic nodal with splenic disease.	Not applicable.
IV	Additional distant extranodal disease.	Not applicable.

Table 4: Ann Arbor classification modified by Cheson et al. Modified from [52].

Specific aspects in initial staging for Hodgkin's lymphoma and Aggressive or Indolent Non-Hodgkin lymphoma:

1. Hodgkin's lymphoma:

Hodgkin's lymphoma accounts for approximately 10% of all lymphomas diagnosed in the industrialized world annually and it is divided into two main types: classical Hodgkin lymphoma and nodular lymphocyte predominance Hodgkin's lymphoma [64]. Hodgkin lymphoma presents, as we have seen, high avidity for 18F-FDG. This entity is usually confined to the lymph nodes at diagnosis and reaches cure rates of 80% [65].

The National Comprehensive Cancer Network indicates that 18F-FDG PET/CT are currently a cornerstone in the initial staging and evaluation of response in the Hodgkin lymphoma [66]. Assessment of response to chemotherapy or combined therapy can be evaluated by interim PET/CT after the 2nd or 4th cycle as well as at the end of treatment, being the persistence of disease at the end of it a negative prognostic factor for disease-free survival [67-68].

Sensitivity and specificity of 18F-FDG to predict disease recurrence are 79% and 97%, respectively, with a negative predictive value greater than 90% in patients with Hodgkin lymphoma after the completion of chemotherapy [69]. In contrast, the positive predictive value is variable, in addition to other false positives such as 18F-FDG increased uptake in post-treatment inflammation, infection, brown fat and the normal physiologic metabolic activity, so the biopsy to confirm the recurrence is mandatory [70].

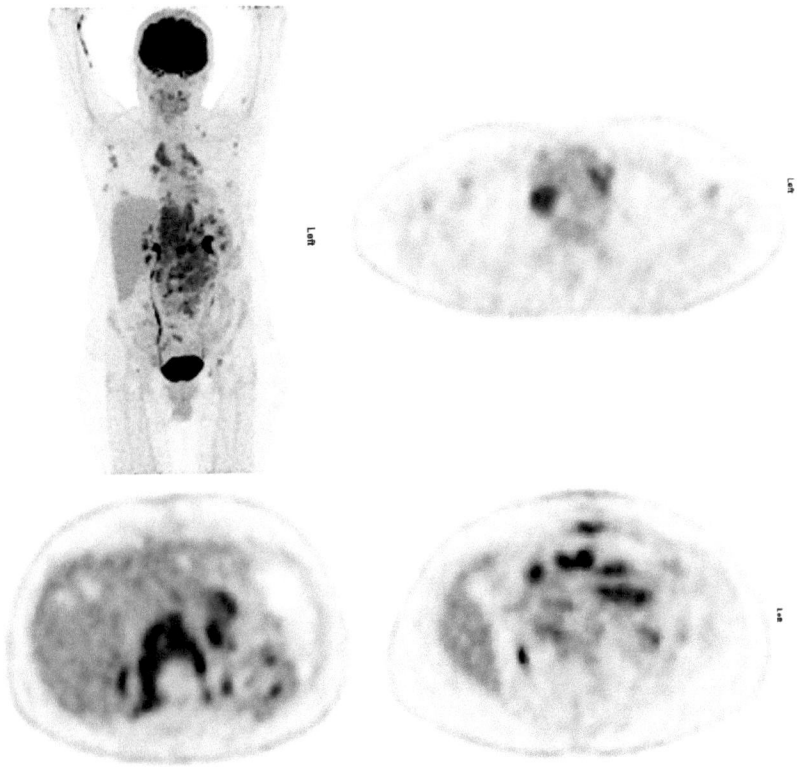

Figure 2: Extensive supra and infra-diaphragmatic lymph node involvement in cervical, axillar, mediastinal (upper right panel), retroperitoneal (lower left panel) and mesenteric adenopathies (lower right panel) in a 41 year old female with diagnostic of follicular lymphoma stage III. A SUV maximum of 8 was measured.

2. Aggressive Non-Hodgkin lymphoma:

Most common types of Non-Hodgkin lymphomas (Diffuse large B-cell lymphoma, Burkitt lymphoma, anaplastic large cell lymphoma), and some indolent lymphoma such as follicular lymphoma are routinely 18F-FDG avid with a sensitivity that exceeds 80% and a specificity of about 90%, which is superior to CT alone [71].

Diffuse large B-cell lymphoma has better documented the role of PET/CT in the initial staging from all of them, because of its higher frequency and rate of avidity for the tracer.

In others as in Burkitt lymphoma, despite its highly FDG-avid, its usefulness in the management is still controversial, although recent papers indicate that PET/CT is a usefulness technique by providing a more accurate staging [72].

However, it has proved useful in establishing accurate staging in patients with Burkitt, anaplastic or mantle cell lymphoma with extranodal involvement [73-76].

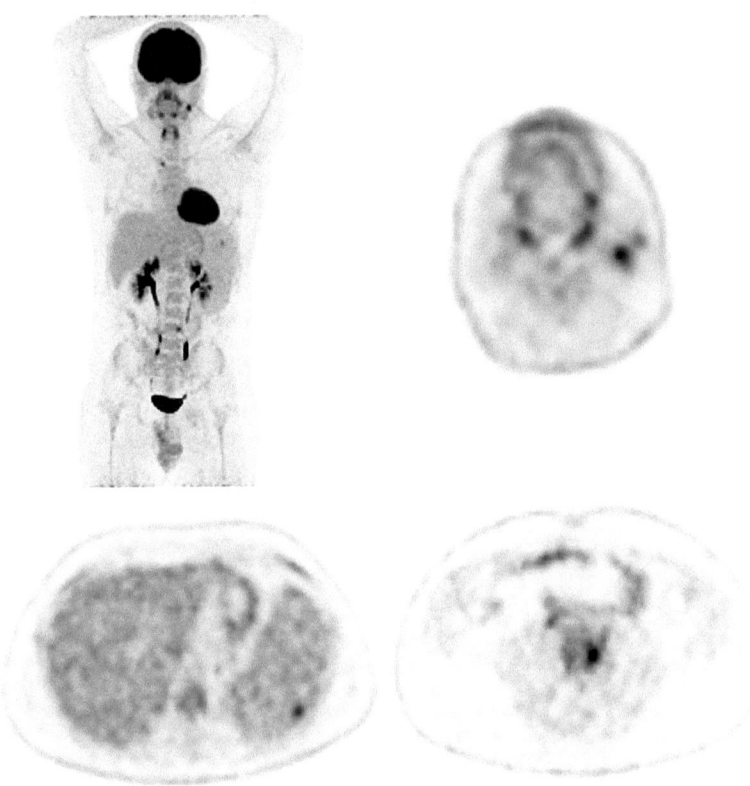

Figure 3: Supradiaphragmatic lymphadenopathies in left retromolar region (upper right panel), lymphomatous splenomegaly (lower left panel) and solitary metabolically positive bone lesion in the L4 body (lower right panel) in a 21 year old male with recent diagnosis of diffuse large B-cell lymphoma stage IV.

3. Indolent Non-Hodgkin lymphoma:

Despite his high avidity for 18F-FDG, PET/CT scanning is not applied for standard staging at diagnosis of follicular lymphoma, being used for assessment of treatment response or when transformation to a high-grade lymphoma is suspected [77].

It is also controversial the use of PET/CT in patients with marginal zone B-cell lymphoma because variability of 18F-FDG avidity. Still, the 18F-FDG PET/CT had showed more involved areas in almost half of patients at diagnosis than with CT alone, and up to 75% of which corresponded to extranodal lesions [78]. Regarding the marginal zone lymphoma of the mucosa-associated lymphoid tissue (MALT), a recent meta-analysis, suggest a potential clinical role of 18F-FDG PET/CT in the initial evaluation because of its high detection rate [79].

There are only a few published papers about the usefulness of PET/CT in staging mycosis fungoides and Sézary syndrome, but it seems that was more sensitive in detecting lymph node involved by lymphoma compared with CT alone data and may provide more accurate staging and prognostic information [80].

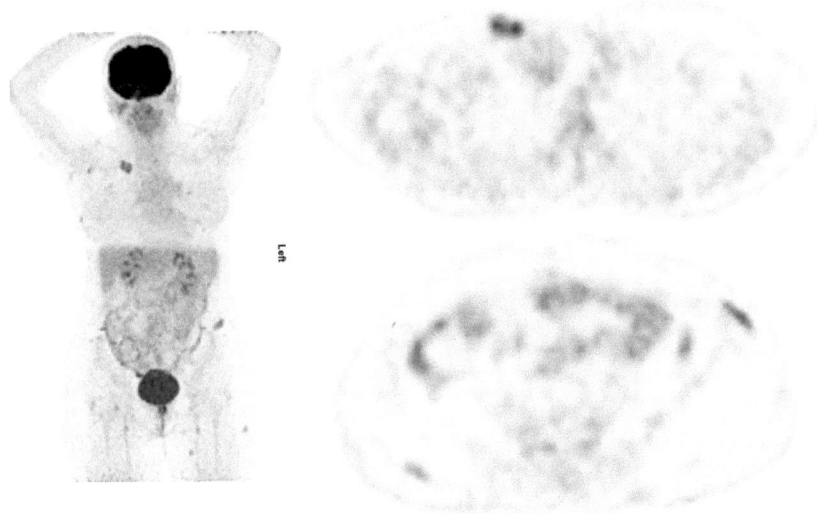

Figure 4: Multiple pathological deposits of 18F-FDG uptake in subcutaneous tissue of trunk and lower limbs, with moderate intensity and SUV maximum of 5.4 in a 52 year old female with diagnosis of marginal zone lymphoma after biopsy of the right breast lesion (upper right panel).

Evaluation of Bone Marrow Involvement:

As we have seen, bone marrow biopsy is a standard method crucial for the evaluation of bone marrow infiltration by lymphoma, giving rise to significant prognostic and therapeutic consequences. However, it is an invasive and painful procedure; so many authors have studied the possibility of using PET/CT to determine the presence or absence of bone marrow disease [81-84].

In this regard, conclusion seems to be that 18F-FDG PET/CT is complementary but could not replace bone marrow biopsy in the evaluation of bone marrow extent, due to the low sensitivity for detection of bone marrow infiltration in lymphoma patients. Nevertheless, allows a whole-body bone marrow examination in addition to being a useful tool for image-guided biopsy for staging lymphoma, especially for aggressive subtypes of Non-Hodgkin lymphoma.

Their main disadvantages are the low rate of detection when it is a located infiltration as well as false positives caused because not every 18F-FDG-avid bone marrow abnormality represents lymphoma [81]. In this sense, a pattern of non-focal, diffusely increased bone marrow 18F-FDG uptake may be related to bone marrow reactivation.

It is known that an early response to chemotherapy is a surrogate marker for chemo-sensitivity in patients with Hodgkin lymphoma and diffuse large B-cell lymphoma, which is associated with increased disease-free survival [85].

In this regard, the 18F-FDG interim PET/CT ensures an early assessment to the response of the established regimen of treatment, once the second or fourth cycle of chemotherapy is completed.

Persistent increased 18F-FDG uptake foci after two or four cycles of chemotherapy are associated with relapses in 50-100% of patients, while relapse is seen in less than 10% of patients with negative findings in the interim PET/CT [86]. Interim PET/CT has a sensitivity of 81% and a specificity of 97% for patients with Hodgkin lymphoma, while it is reaching levels of 78% and 87% respectively, for patients with diffuse large B-cell lymphoma [87].

Regarding patients with indolent lymphomas, there is still little evidence to support the use of 18F-FDG interim PET/CT for monitoring the treatment response [88], because of their lower avidity for the tracer.

Currently, 18F-FDG interim PET/CT studies are read according to visual criteria, being the definition of a positive interim-PET result has evolved from any uptake above background to an intensity exceeding the background in the liver [89]. The current criteria for the assessment of interim PET/CT is the Deauville 5-point scale that provides a flexible reading scheme suitable for different positivity thresholds. Table 5 summarizes the Deauville criteria.

Score	Grade of 18F-FDG uptake
1	No uptake
2	Uptake ≤ mediastinum
3	Uptake > mediastinum and ≤ liver
4	Uptake moderately increased above liver
5	Markedly increased uptake above liver and/or new sites of disease

Table 5: Visual assessment of 18F-FDG uptake at interim PET/CT according to Deauville criteria. Modified from [47].

18F-FDG PET/CT is superior to CT alone to assess early response. Concerning the modification of the established treatment regimen (in the sense of limiting the number of cycles in responding patients or to switch to more aggressive schemes in non-responders ones), trials are evaluating the role of PET response–adapted therapy. Currently, changing treatment solely on the basis of 18F-FDG interim PET/CT is not recommended, unless there is clear evidence of progression [60, 90].

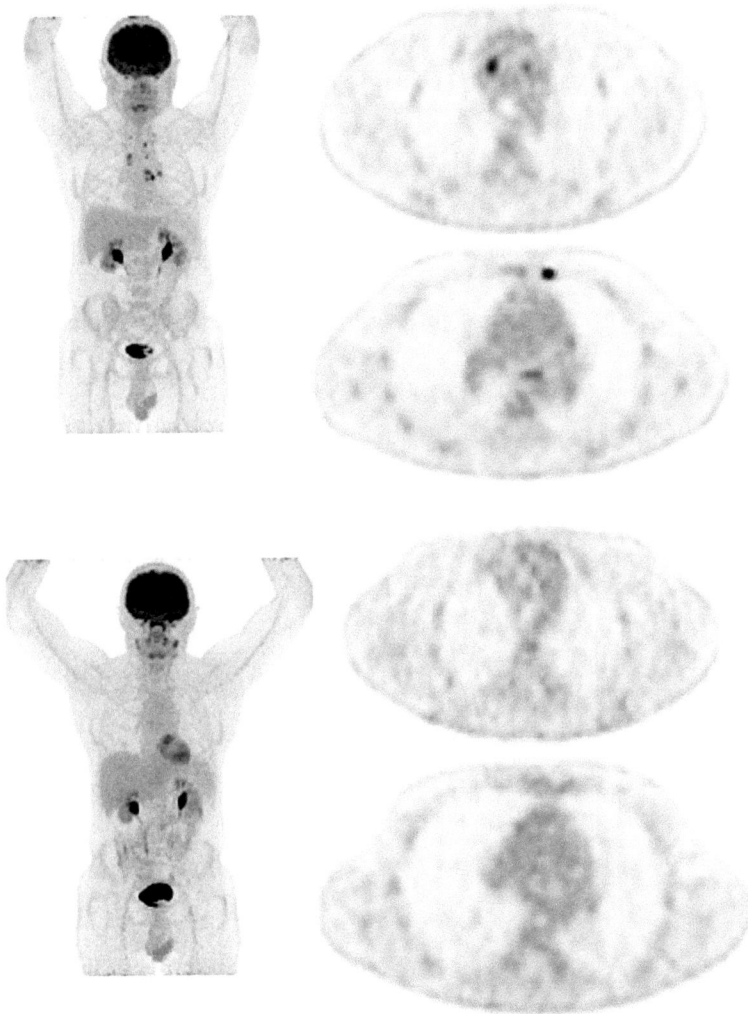

Figure 5: Initial staging PET/CT (above) revealing hypermetabolic lymphadenopathy with high rate of cell proliferation in the mediastinum and left internal mammary chain in a 42 year old male with diagnosis of Hodgkin lymphoma. Interim 18F-FDG PET/CT (below) is demonstrating of complete metabolic response after 2 cycles of chemotherapy.

PET/CT in the assessment of final response to treatment

18F-FDG PET/CT is the standard of care for remission assessment in 18F-FDG-avid lymphoma because of its ability to distinguish fibrosis or sclerosis from residual active disease.

Although 18F-FDG PET/CT was considered standard for staging since 2007 guidelines, visual interpretation is still used; conditioning that inter-observer variability also remains a problem [91]. The actually accepted scale for evaluating studies at the end of treatment is summarized in Table 6.

The standardization of PET/CT methods is desirable for best clinical practice. In this regard, PET/CT after completion of therapy should be performed preferably at 6-8 weeks after chemotherapy or chemo-immunotherapy, and 8-12 weeks after radiation or chemoradiotherapy according with NCCN recommendations [91].

The presence of residual metabolically active tissue at the end of therapy in patients with Hodgkin lymphoma and diffuse large B-cell lymphoma, a biopsy is recommended when considering salvage therapy [47].

In patients who have received salvage therapy with stem cell transplantation, post-salvage therapy 18F-FDG PET/CT is also recommended to differentiate patients with a better prognosis from others with unfavorable prognosis [90].

Response criteria	Definition
Complete remission	Disappearance of all evidence of disease. Score 1, 2, or 3 (5-point scale) with or without a residual mass. Lymph nodes/masses must regress to ≤1.5 cm in largest diameter. No evidence of extranodal involvement.
Partial remission	Score 4 or 5 with reduced uptake compared with baseline PET/CT. Decrease ≥50% in the sum of the maximum diameters of lymphatic and spleen involvement.
Stable disease	Score 4 or 5 with no significant changes from baseline PET/CT. <50% decrease in the sum of the maximum diameters of lesions.
Progressive disease	Score 4, 5 with an increase in intensity of uptake from baseline and/or new FDG-avid foci, >1.5 cm in any axis, consistent with lymphoma at interim or end of treatment PET/CT.

Table 6: 18F-FDG PET/CT response score at the end of the treatment. Modified from [47].

PET/CT in the routine follow-up of lymphoma

Surveillance imaging of asymptomatic patients with lymphoma once observed remission of the disease remains controversial because it offers little clinical benefit [92]. Routine follow-up 18F-FDG PET/CT was also associated with a high rate of false positives, mainly due to reactive lymphadenitis and/or granulomatosis. For patients with a positive PET and a negative CT, the false-positive rate was 42% [93]. All this becomes the scan a not very cost-effective technique [92].

In up to 80% of cases, is the patient or the doctor who identified the recurrence before it is detected by routine imaging studies [93]. Relapse in patients with Hodgkin lymphoma appears often as clinically silent disease. This may explain why the 18F-FDG PET/CT may be superior to clinical examination. However, its earlier diagnosis is not associated with improved survival [90]. In other hand, routine follow-up scanning in patients with indolent lymphoma is not justified [93].

In summary, the low positive predictive value associated with routine follow-up 18F-FDG PET/CT scans denies their clinical value in identifying patients who would benefit from additional treatment [93].

Chapter 3

Primary adrenal lymphoma and nuclear medicine

Introduction

Primary adrenal lymphoma (PAL) is a histologically proven lymphoma that involves one or both adrenal glands. In this entity, at presentation there is no prior history of lymphoma elsewhere and, if lymph nodes or other organs are involved, adrenal lesions are unequivocally dominant [95]. Here, when there is extranodal involvement, usually it affects the CNS and the GI tract, as well as other endocrine organs [96]. This entity is extremely rare accounting for less than 1% of all non-Hodgkin's lymphoma cases and 3% of extranodal lymphoma [97, 98]. Histologically, the most common subtype is diffuse large B-cell lymphoma (75%) followed by peripheral T-cell lymphoma and Hodgkin disease [99]. The male/female ratio is 3:1, primarily affecting elderly men at about 60 years [100]. About 70% of PAL are bilateral and the most common presenting symptoms are fever of unknown origin, asthenia, abdominal pain, constipation and adrenal failure [97, 101, 102]. The ethiopathology is unknown but Epstein-Barr Virus, immune dysfunction as autoinmune disease, mutations in the *p53* and *c-kit* genes, concurrent or past history of cancer and human immunodeficiency virus infection have been implicated [102-104]. PAL should always be considered in differential diagnosis of bilateral adrenal mass with adrenal insufficiency [105-106].

For diagnosis, on CT and magnetic resonance imaging, PALs tend to appear as complex masses of variable density and often have areas of necrosis and/or hemorrhage [107]. Magnetic resonance imaging (MRI) allows for the detection of adrenal masses with a similar sensitivity as CT but is not considered quite as accurate as CT. However, MRI may be useful in ambiguous cases [108, 109].

PAL is a very rare entity and to date there is no defined treatment protocol. Most patients are treated with regimens similar to those used to treat other types of lymphoma. Therapeutic modalities proposed are inmunochemotherapy, surgery, radiotherapy, steroid replacement and intrathecal profilaxis [99, 103, 110]. The most common regimen of PAL is R-CHOP (Rituximab-Cyclophosphamide, Dorubicin,

39

Vincristine, Prednisone), which has been proposed as the first-line treatment in this entity. Kim YR, et al [111] reported complete remission and overall response rate of 54.8% and 87%, respectively, in 31 patients diagnosed with primary adrenal diffuse large B-cell lymphoma and treated with a median 6 cycles of R-CHOP chemotherapy. In patients achieving complete remission, significant prolongations of overall survival (OS) (p = 0.029) and progression-free survival (PFS) (p = 0.005) were observed. The 2-year estimates of OS and PFS were 68.3% and 51.1%, respectively. On the other hand, patients with PAL reminder have been treated with CVP or MACCOP-B [112]. Radiotherapy is also used, but in a very limited number of cases, however, the results appear to be ineffectual [113]. When there is adrenal insufficiency, hormone replacement therapy is mandatory.

The prognosis is poor with a median survival of 12.5 weeks despite aggressive chemotherapy, especially when there are secondary SNC involvement which occurs in 2-10% of all cases of diffuse large B-cell lymphoma [106]. Prognostic and risk factors include age, elevated serum LDH levels, adrenal insufficiency at time of presentation and involvement of multiple extranodal sites [114, 115].

Historical background

In the past, whole body gallium (67Ga) scan was used as a baseline for staging, to assess gallium avidity, and to assess the response to therapy of Hodgkin's lymphoma and non-Hodgkin lymphoma, as well as PAL [114-116].

Truong B et al [114] reported the case of a 38-year-old male with fever, night sweats and weight lost. After physical exam, the CT scan revealed a heterogeneous low-density left suprarenal mass displacing the left kidney. Subsequently, histological examination of the core needle biopsy revealed large B-cell lymphoma. Moreover, a whole body 67-gallium (67Ga) scan was performed showing a large area of intense radiotracer accumulation in the left upper quadrant, which correlated with the CT findings. With this finding, the diagnosis of PAL was made. The patient initiated aggressive chemotherapy and follow-up CT and gallium scan showed decrease in size and uptake of radiotracer in the region of tumor. Then, consolidation radiotherapy was administered.

PET/CT role in the present context

Currently, the whole body 67-gallium (67Ga) scan has been relegated by 18F-FDG PET/CT due to its higher accuracy in the detection of both entities and the much better quality of the images provided by this diagnostic tool, as has been discussed in the previous chapter.

18F-FDG PET/CT has proven to be a powerful tool in tumor diagnosis and staging, monitoring response to treatment, and detecting recurrence of Hodgkin's and non-Hodgkin's lymphoma. Furthermore, follow-up scans may be considered in indolent lymphomas with residual intra-abdominal or retroperitoneal disease [117]. In addition, as the adrenal lesions, 18F-FDG PET/CT is an important imaging modality for characterization, and particularly for PAL. In this regard, it has been reported that adrenocortical carcinomas and PAL often show moderate to severe 18F-FDG uptake [105]. There are few studies on PAL and nuclear medicine, and most are case reports.

Martínez-Esteve A et al [75] reported the case of a 71-year-old male patient with weight loss, hypotension and fatigue. The contrast-enhanced CT showed two large bilateral adrenal masses producing displacement of the renal poles and the splenic vein. Subsequent biopsy showed diffuse large B-cell lymphoma and the initial staging 18F-FDG PET/CT evidenced intense 18F-FDG uptake by the adrenal masses with a maximum standardized uptake value (SUVmax) of 24.6, and with no evidence of extra-adrenal spread (Figure 6). With these findings, the patient was treated with 6 cycles of R-CHOP chemotherapy. A post-treatment 18F-FDG PET/CT showed the disappearance of the pathological 18F-FDG uptake in the adrenal region (SUVmax of 3.5), suggesting a likely complete metabolic response (Figure 7).

Kim KM, et al. [105] reported the case of a 52-year-old man with blood pressure 100/70 mmHg, body temperature 38.5°C, and laboratory tests showing changes suggesting adrenal insufficiency (LDH 476 IU/l, serum cortisol concentration at 8 am 2.9 µg/dl, plasma ACTH level at 8 am 210 pg/ml, serum aldosterone concentration 56.2 pg/ml). CT scan showed large bilateral adrenal masses (right adrenal gland 5.8 x 2.7 cm, and the left adrenal gland 3.7 x 2 cm). After CT-guided core needle biopsy of the adrenal mass, the tumor was diagnosed as diffuse large B-cell lymphoma. 18F-FDG PET/CT demonstrated intense FDG accumulation in both adrenal glands, with no abnormal FDG uptake in the rest of the body. For treatment, the patient was administered adrenal hormone replacement therapy, and also administered 6 cycles of R-CHOP chemotherapy. No evidence of tumor on follow-up 18F-FDG PET/CT scan.

These two cases demonstrate the importance of performing an 18F-FDG PET/CT study to monitor response to treatment in PAL, as already described in previous studies in Hodgkin and non-Hodgkin lymphoma [118-120].

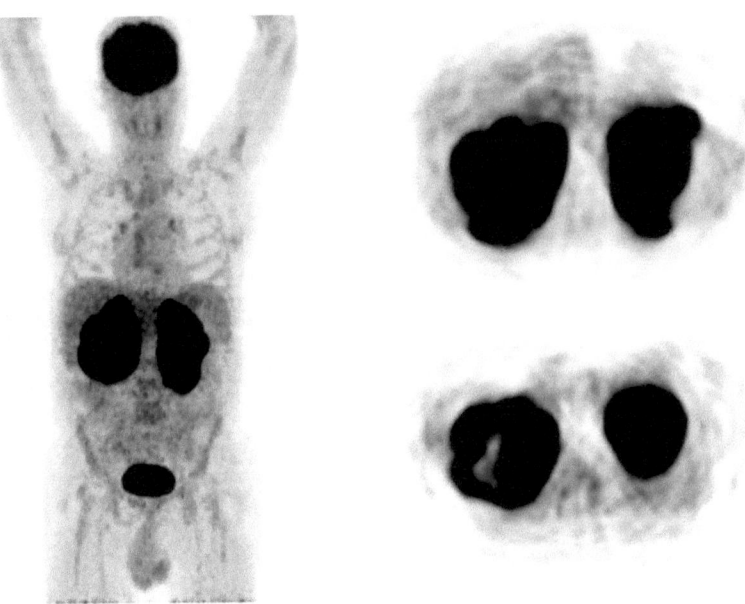

Figure 6: Maximum intensity projection and axial images of a staging 18F-FDG PET/CT study showing large adrenal masses with intense FDG uptake (SUVmax of 24.6), without evidence of extra-adrenal spread, in a 71-year-old male with primary bilateral diffuse large-B cell lymphoma of the adrenals [75].

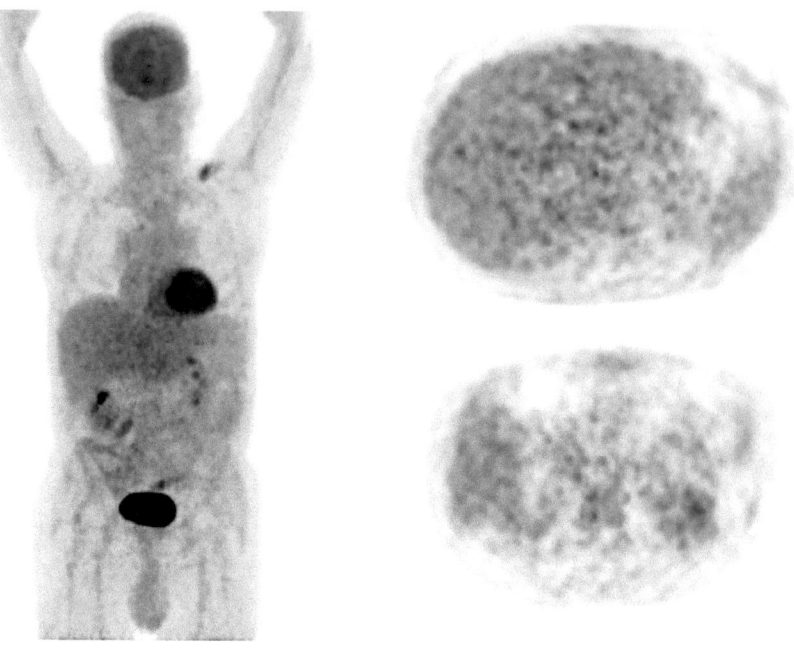

Figure 7: Images after 6 cycles of R-CHOP chemotherapy. Maximum intensity projection and axial images of a monitoring treatment 18F-FDG PET/CT study showing no evidence of tumor in the adrenal region (SUVmax of 3.5).

Ozimek A, et al [121] reported the case of a 84-year-old male patient with a six-moth history of significant weight loss and lumbar pain. Contrast-enhanced CT scan revealed splenomegaly and large bilateral adrenal masses without abdominal lymphadenopathy. Subsequent 18F-FDG PET/CT showed an intense FDG accumulation in both adrenal glands without abnormal FDG uptake in extraadrenal regions. Due to de large diameter of the two masses were highly suggestive of malignancy, open bilateral adrenalectomy was performed. Histopahological examination revealed diffuse large B-cell lymphoma. Adjuvant cyclophosphamide, dorubicin, vincristine, prednisone (CHOP) scheme was started. However, the patient died during follow-up because of disseminated progressive disease and cardiopulmonary failure.

Kübra Aydin, et al [122] reported the case of a 75-year-old male with dullness for duration of 2 months. A brain MRI revealed a paramedian subcortical mass measuring 30 x 25 x 25 mm located on the superior and middle frontal gyrus of the left brain hemisphere. In addition, a mass was observed at the right frontal periventricular. Surgical intervention and excisional biopsy revealed a CD20+ large B cell lymphoma. After physical examination and laboratory tests, the patient underwent 18F-FDG PET/CT which revealed a FDG uptake focus only in the adrenal glands, without glycolytic activity in the brain and other regions of the body. A CT-guided fine needle aspiration biopsy revealed a CD20+ large B cell lymphoma similar in presentation to the patient's brain pathology. The patient was treated with whole-brain radiotherapy and subsequent chemotherapy (R-CHOP). However, the patient died at the end of 6 months of follow-up period due to disease progression.

References

1. Shankland KR, Armitage JO, Hancock BW. Non-Hodgkin lymphoma. The Lancet. 2012;380:848-857.

2. Ferlay J, Steliarova-Foucher E, Lortet-Tieulent J, et al. Cancer incidence and mortality patterns in Europe: estimates for 40 countries in 2012. Eur J Cancer. 2013;49:1374-403.

3. Bray F, Ren JS, Masuyer E, et al. Estimates of global cancer prevalence for 27 sites in the adult population in 2008. Int J Cancer. 2013;132:1133-45.

4. EER stat fact sheets: non-Hogkin lymphoma. Bethesda, Maryland, US: National Cancer Institute, National Institutes of Health. Information published online, accessed May 2015.

5. Leukemia and Lymphoma Society, Facts 2015-2015, accessed June 2015.

6. Feldman AL, Pittaluga S, Jaffe ES. Classification and histopatologhy of lymphomas. In: Canellos GP, Lister TA, Young BD (Ed). The Lymphomas (Second Edition). Philadelphia, USA: Saunders Elsevier; 2006. pp: 2-38.

7. Swerdlow SH, Campo E, Harris NL, et al. WHO Classification of Tumours of Haematopoietic and Lymphoid Tissues. Lyon, France: IARC Press; 2008.

8. Campo E, Swerdlow SH, Harris NL, et al. The 2008 WHO classification of lymphoid neoplasms and beyond: evolving concepts and practical applications. Blood. 2011;117:5019-5032.

9. Küppers R, Engert A, Hansmann ML. Hodgkin lymphoma. J Clin Invest. 2012;122:3439-3447.

10. Kapatai G, Murray P. Contribution of the Epstein Barr virus to the molecular pathogenesis of Hodgkin lymphoma. J Clin Pathol. 2007;60:1342-1349.

11. Engert A, Horning SJ. Hodgkin Lymphoma. Heidelberg, Germany: Springer; 2011.

12. PDQ Adult Treatment Editorial Board. Adult Non-Hodgkin Lymphoma Treatment (PDQ®): Health Professional Version. PDQ Cancer Information Summaries [Internet]. Bethesda (MD): National Cancer Institute (US); 2002-. 2015 Aug 7.

13. Ansell SM, Armitage J. Non-Hodgkin lymphoma: diagnosis and treatment. Mayo Clin Proc. 2005;80:1087-97.

14. Salvatore JR, Ross RS. Primary bilateral adrenal lymphoma. Leuk Lymphoma. 1999;34:111-7.

15. Winn J, Stock H. Primary lymphoma of bone. Conn Med. 2015;79:173-5.

16. Simpson WG, Lopez A, Babbar P, et al. Primary bladder lymphoma diffuse large B-cell type: Case report and literature review of 26 cases. 2015;7:268-72.

17. Zhou HY, Gao F, Bu B, et al. Primary bone lymphoma: A case report and review of the literature. Oncol Lett. 2014;8:1551-6.

18. Dolecek TA, Propp JM, Stroup NE, et al. CBTRUS statistical report: Primary brain and central nervous system tumors diagnosed in the United States in 2005–2009. Neuro Oncol. 2012;14.

19. Lloyd IE, Clement PW, Salzman KL, et al. An unusual and challenging case of HIV-associated primary CNS lymphoma with Hodgkin-like morphology and HIV encephalitis. Diagn Pathol. 2015;10:152.

20. Phillips EH, Fox CP. Primary CNS lymphoma. Curr Hematol Malig Rep. 2014;9:243-53.

21. Weller M, Martus P, Roth P, et al. Surgery for primary CNS Lymphoma? Challenging a paradigm. Neuro Oncol. 2012;14:1481–4.

22. Kawai N, Miyake K, Yamamoto Y, et al. 18FFDG PET in the diagnosis and treatment of primary central nervous system lymphoma. Biomed Res Int. 2013;2013:247152.

23. Thiel E, Korfel A, Martus P, et al. High-dose methotrexate with or without whole brain radiotherapy for primary CNS lymphoma (G-PCNSL-SG-1): a phase 3, randomised, non-inferiority trial. Lancet Oncol. 2010;11:1036-47.

24. Zinzani PL, Magagnoli M, Pagliani G, et al. Primary intestinal lymphoma: clinical and therapeutic features of 32 patients. 1997;82:305-8.

25. Vetro C, Bonanno G, Giulietti G, et al. Rare gastrointestinal lymphomas: The endoscopic investigation. World J Gastrointest Endosc. 2015;7:928-49.

26. Graham RL, Mardones MA, Krause JR. Primary follicular lymphoma of the duodenum. Proc (Bayl Univ Med Cent). 2015;28:381-3.

27. Zhang S, Wang L, Yu D, et al. Localized primary gastrointestinal diffuse large B cell lymphoma received a surgical approach: an analysis of prognostic factors and comparison of staging systems in 101 patients from a single institution. World J Surg Oncol. 2015;13:246.

28. Paras CA, Salpin AP, Veloso JD. Primary thyroid lymphoma. Philipp J Otolaryngol Head Neck Surg. 2012;27:38-40.

29. Li XB, Ye ZX. Primary thyroid lymphoma: multi-slice computed tomography findings. Asian Pac J Cancer Prev. 2015;16:1135-8.

30. Verma D, Puri V, Agarwal S, et al. Primary thyroid lymphoma: A rare disease. J Cytol. 2014;31:218-20.

31. Horasanli K, Kadihasanoglu M, Aksakal OT, et al. A case of primary lymphoma of the bladder managed with multimodal therapy. Nat Clin Pract Urol. 2008;5:167-70.

32. Simpson WG, Lopez A, Babbar P, et al. Primary bladder lymphoma, diffuse large B-cell type: Case report and literature review of 26 cases. Urol Ann. 2015;7:268-72.

33. Maninderpal KG, Amir FH, Azad HA, et al. Imaging findings of a primary bladder maltoma. Br J Radiol. 2011;84:e186-90.

34. Zhou HY, Gao F, Bu B, et al. Primary bone lymphoma: A case report and review of the literature. Oncol Lett. 2014;8:1551-6.

35. Beal K, Allen L, Yahalom J. Primary bone lymphoma: treatment results and prognostic factors with long-term follow-up of 82 patients. Cancer. 2006;106: 2652-6.

36. Lewis VO, Primus G, Anastasi J, et al. Oncologic outcomes of primary lymphoma of bone in adults. Clin Orthop Relat Res. 2003;415:90-7.

37. Wang LJ, Wu HB, Wang M, et al. Utility of F-18 FDG PET/CT on the evaluation of primary bone lymphoma. Eur J Radiol. 2015. pii: S0720-048X(15)30103-0 doi: 10.1016/j.ejrad.2015.09.011.

38. Park YH, Kim S, Choi SJ, et al. Clinical impact of whole-body FDG-PET for evaluation of response and therapeutic decision-making of primary lymphoma of bone. Ann Oncol. 2005;16:1401-2.

39. Ramadan KM, Shenkier T, Sehn LH, et al. A clinicopathological retrospective study of 131 patients with primary bone lymphoma: a population-based study of successively treated cohorts from the British Columbia Cancer Agency. Ann Oncol. 2007;18:129-35

40. Rosenberg SA, Boiron M, De Vita VT Jr, et al. Report of the Committee on Hodgkin's Disease Staging Procedures. Cancer Res 1971;31:1862-1863.

41. Fishman EK, Kuhlman JE, Jones RJ. CT of lymphoma: spectrum of disease. Radiographics 1991;11:647e69.

42. Howell SJ, Grey M, Chang J, et al. The value of bone marrow examination in the staging of Hodgkin's lymphoma: a review of 955 cases seen in a regional cancer centre. Br J Haematol 2002;119:408e11.

43. Vassilakopoulos TP, Angelopoulou MK, Constantinou N, et al. Development and validation of a clinical prediction rule for bone marrow involvement in patients with Hodgkin lymphoma. Blood 2005;105:1875e80.

44. Delbeke D, Stroobants S, De Kerviler E, et al. Expert opinions on positron emission tomography and computed tomography imaging in lymphoma. Oncologist. 2009;14:30-40.

45. Cabrera A, Gámez C, Martín JC. Tomografía por emisión de positrones (PET) en oncología clínica. Rev Esp Med Nuclear. 2002;21:131–47.

46. Podoloff DA, Advani RH, Allred C, et al. NCCN task force report: positron emission tomography (PET)/computed tomography (CT) scanning in cancer. J Natl Compr Canc Netw. 2007;5:S1–22.

47. Wang X. PET/CT: appropriate application in lymphoma. Chin Clin Oncol. 2015:4:4.

48. Weiler-Sagie M, Bushelev O, Epelbaum R, et al. 18F-FDG Avidity in Lymphoma Readdressed: A Study of 766 Patients. J Nucl Med. 2010; 51:25-30.

49. Baba S, Abe K, Isoda T, et al. Impact of FDG-PET/CT in the management of lymphoma. Ann Nucl Med. 2011;25:701-16.

50. Álvarez Páez AM, Nogueiras Alonso JM, Serena Puig A. 18F-FDG-PET/TC en linfoma: dos décadas de experiencia. Rev Esp Med Nucl Imagen Mol. 2012;31(6):340–349.

51. Schöder H, Noy A, Gönen M, et al. Intensity of 18fluorodeoxyglucose uptake in positron emission tomography distinguishes between indolent and aggressive non-Hodgkin's lymphoma. J Clin Oncol. 2005;23:4643–51.

52. Cheson BD, Fisher RI, Barrington SF, et al: Recommendations for initial evaluation, staging, and response assessment of Hodgkin and nonHodgkin lymphoma: The Lugano classification. J Clin Oncol. 2014;32:3059-3068.

53. Herrmann K, Buck AK, Schuster T, et al: Week one FLT-PET response predicts complete remission to R-CHOP and survival in DLBCL. Oncotarget. 2014;5:4050-4059.

54. Herrmann K, Buck AK, Schuster T, et al: A pilot study to evaluate 3'-deoxy-3'-18F-fluorothymidine pet for initial and early response imaging in mantle cell lymphoma. J Nucl Med. 2011;52:1898-1902.

55. Li Z, Graf N, Herrmann K, et al: FLT-PET is superior to FDG-PET for very early response prediction in NPM-ALK-positive lymphoma treated with targeted therapy. Cancer Res. 2012;72:5014-5024.

56. Mena E, Lindenberg ML, Turkbey BI, et al: A pilot study of the value of 18 F-fluoro-deoxy-thymidine PET/CT in predicting viable lymphoma in residual 18F-FDG avid masses after completion of therapy. Clin Nucl Med. 2014;39:874-881.

57. Dhilly M, Guillouet S, Patin D, et al: 2-[18F]fludarabine, a novel positron emission tomography (PET) tracer for imaging lymphoma: A micro-PET study in murine models. Mol Imaging Biol. 2014;16:118-126.

58. Cheson BD, Pfistner B, Juweid ME, et al: Revised response criteria for malignant lymphoma. J Clin Oncol. 2007; 25:579-586.

59. Barrington SF, Mackewn JE, Schleyer P, et al: Establishment of a UK-wide network to facilitate the acquisition of quality assured FDG-PET data for clinical trials in lymphoma. Ann Oncol. 2011; 22:739-745.

60. Barrington SF, Mikhaeel NG, Kostakoglu L, et al: Role of imaging in the staging and response assessment of lymphoma: Consensus of the International Conference on Malignant Lymphomas Imaging Working Group. J Clin Oncol. 2014;32:3048-58.

61. Saboo SS, Krajewski KM, O'Regan KN, et al: Spleen in haematological malignancies: Spectrum of imaging findings. Br J Radiol. 2012; 85:81-92.

62. Abrey LE, Batchelor TT, Ferreri AJ, et al: Report of an international workshop to standardize baseline evaluation and response criteria for primary CNS lymphoma. J Clin Oncol. 2005;23:5034-5043

63. Zucca E, Copie-Bergman C, Ricardi U, et al: Gastric marginal zone lymphoma of MALT type: ESMO Clinical Practice Guidelines for diagnosis, treatment, and follow-up. Ann Oncol. 2013; 24:vi144-vi148.

64. Jemal A, Siegel R, Ward E, et al. Cancer statistics, 2009. CA Cancer J. Clin. 2009;59:225-249.

65. Siegel R, Naishadham D, Jemal A. Cancer statistics, 2013. CA Cancer J. Clin. 2013;63:11-30.

66. Keraliya AR, Tirumani SH, Shinagare AB, et al. Beyond PET/CT in Hodgkin lymphoma: a comprehensive review of the role of imaging at initial presentation, during follow-up and for assessment of treatment-related complications. Insights Imaging. 2015;6:381-92.

67. de Wit M, Bohuslavizki KH, Buchert R, et al. 18FDG-PET following treatment as valid predictor for disease-free survival in Hodgkin's lymphoma. Ann Oncol Off J Euro Soc Med Oncol/ ESMO. 2001;12:29–37.

68. Naumann R, Vaic A, Beuthien-Baumann B, et al. Prognostic value of positron emission tomography in the evaluation of post-treatment residual mass in patients with Hodgkin's disease and non-Hodgkin's lymphoma. Br J Haematol. 2001;115:793–800.

69. Guay C, Lepine M, Verreault J, et al. Prognostic value of PET using 18 F-FDG in Hodgkin's disease for posttreatment evaluation. J Nuc Med Off Pub Soc Nuc Med. 2003; 44:1225–1231.

70. El-Galaly TC, Mylam KJ, Brown P, et al. Positron emission tomography/computed tomography surveillance in patients with Hodgkin lymphoma in first remission has a low positive predictive value and high costs. Haematologica. 2012; 97:931–936.

71. Buchmann I, Reinhardt M, Elsner K, et al. 2-(fluorine-18) fluoro-2-deoxy-D-glucose positron emission tomography in the detection and staging of malignant lymphoma: a bicenter trial. Cancer 2001;91:889-899.

72. Carrillo-Cruz E, Marín-Oyaga VA, Solé Rodríguez M, et al. Role of 18F-FDG-PET/CT in the management of Burkitt lymphoma. Eur J Haematol. 2015;94:23-30.

73. Uslu L, Sen F, Sager S, et al. Extensive peritoneal and pleural lymphomatosis in a patient with Burkitt lymphoma revealed with 18F-FDG PET/CT. Nuklearmedizin. 2013; 52:N56-7.

74. Granero PJ, Gómez FJ, Mercado MR, et al. 18F-FDG PET/CT in Extranodal Burkitt Lymphoma. Clin Nucl Med. 2015 Jun 19. [Epub ahead of print]

75. Martínez-Esteve A, García-Gómez FJ, Borrero-Martin JJ, et al. 18F-FDG PET/CT in a case of bilateral lacrimal gland infiltration by mantle cell lymphoma. Rev Esp Med Nucl Imagen Mol. 2015 May 5. pii: S2253-654X(15)00033-5. doi: 10.1016/j.remn.2015.03.006.

76. Acevedo-Báñez I, García-Gomez FJ, Jiménez-Granero P, et al. 18F-FDG-PET/CT in implant-associated anaplastic large cell lymphoma of the breast. Br J Haematol. 2015;169:1.

77. Novelli S, Briones J, Flotats A, et al. ET/CT Assessment of Follicular Lymphoma and High Grade B Cell Lymphoma – Good Correlation with Clinical and Histological Features at Diagnosis. Adv Clin Exp Med. 2015;24:325-330.

78. Carrillo-Cruz E, Marín-Oyaga VA, de la Cruz Vicente F, et al. Role of 18F-FDG-PET/CT in the management of marginal zone B cell lymphoma. Hematol Oncol. 2014 Nov 19. doi: 10.1002/hon.2181.

79. Treglia G, Zucca E, Sadeghi R, et al. Detection rate of fluorine-18-fluorodeoxyglucose positron emission tomography in patients with marginal zone lymphoma of MALT type: a meta-analysis. Hematol Oncol. 2014 Jul 22. doi: 10.1002/hon.2152.

80. Tsai EY, Taur A, Espinosa L, et al. Staging accuracy in mycosis fungoides and sezary syndrome using integrated positron emission tomography and computed tomography. Arch Dermatol. 2006;142:577-84.

81. Adams HJA, Nievelstein RAJ, Kwee TC. Opportunities and limitations of bone marrow biopsy and bone marrow FDG-PET in lymphoma. Blood Rev (2015), http://dx.doi.org/10.1016/j.blre.2015.06.003

82. Kim HY, Kim JS, Choi DR, et al. The Clinical Utility of FDG PET-CT in Evaluation of Bone Marrow Involvement by Lymphoma. Cancer Res Treat. 2014 Nov 24. doi: 10.4143/crt.2014.091.

83. Muzahir S, Mian M, Munir I, et al. Clinical utility of ^{18}F FDG-PET/CT in the detection of bone marrow disease in Hodgkin's lymphoma. Br J Radiol. 2012;85:e490-6.

84.   Zhou Z, Chen C, Li X, et al. Evaluation of bone marrow involvement in extranodal NK/T cell lymphoma by FDG-PET/CT. Ann Hematol. 2015;94:963-7.

85.   Haw R, Sawka CA, Franssen E, et al. Significance of a partial or slow response to frontline chemotherapy in the management of intermediate-grade or high-grade non-Hodgkin's lymphoma: a literature review. J Clin Oncol. 1994; 12:1074-84.

86.   Gallamini A, Hutchings M, Rigacci L, et al. Early interim 2-[18F]fluoro-2-deoxy-d-glucose positron emission tomography is prognostically superior to international prognostic score in advancedstage Hodgkin's lymphoma: a report from a joint Italian-Danish study. J Clin Oncol. 2007;25:3746-52.

87.   Terasawa T, Lau J, Bardet S, et al. Fluorine-18-fluorodeoxyglucose positron emission tomography for interim response assessment of advanced stage Hodgkin's lymphoma and diffuse large B-cell lymphoma: a systematic review. J Clin Oncol. 2009;27:1906-14.

88.   Hutchings M, Barrington SF. PET/CT for therapy response assessment in lymphoma. J Nucl Med. 2009;50 Suppl 1:21S-30S.

89.   Barrington SF, Qian W, Somer EJ, et al. Concordance between four European centres of PET reporting criteria designed for use in multicentre trials in Hodgkin lymphoma. Eur J Nucl Med Mol Imaging. 2010;37:1824–33.

90.   Kostakoglu L, Cheson BD. State-of-the-Art Research on "Lymphomas: Role of Molecular Imaging for Staging, Prognostic Evaluation, and Treatment Response". Front Oncol. 2013;3:212.

91.   Zanoni L, Cerci JJ, Fanti S. Use of PET/CT to evaluate response to therapy in lymphoma. Q J Nucl Med Mol Imaging. 2011;55:633-47.

92.   Huntington SF, Svoboda J, Doshi JA. Cost-effectiveness analysis of routine surveillance imaging of patients with diffuse large B-cell lymphoma in first remission. J Clin Oncol. 2015;33:1467-74.

93.   Cheson B. The case against heavy PETing. J Clin Oncol. 2009;27:1742-3.

94.   Rashidi A, Fisher SI. Primary adrenal lymphoma: a systematic review. Ann Hematol. 2013;92:1583–93.

95. Salvatore JR, Ross RS. Primary bilateral adrenal lymphoma. Leuk Lymphoma. 1999;34:111-7.

96. Singh D, Kumar L, Sharma A, et al. Adrenal involvement in non-Hodgkin's lymphoma: four cases and review of literature. Leuk Lymphoma 2004;45:789–94.

97. Freeman C, Berg JW, Culter SJ. Occurrence and prognosis of extranodal lymphomas. Cancer. 1972:29:252-60.

98. Kim SH, Brennan MF, Russo P, et al. The role of surgery in the treatment of clinically isolated adrenal metastasis. Cancer. 1998;82:389-94.

99. Ellis RD, Read D. Bilateral adrenal non-Hodgkin's lymphoma with adrenal insufficiency. Postgrad Med J. 2000;76:508-9.

100. Wang J, Sun NC, Renslo R, et al. Clinically silent primary adrenal lymphoma: a case report and review of the literature. Am J Hematol. 1998;58:130-6.

101. Ohsawa M, Tomita Y, Hashimoto M, et al. Malignant lymphoma of the adrenal gland: its possible correlation with the Epstein-Barr virus. Mod Pathol. 1996;9:534-43.

102. Nakatsuka S, Hongyo T, Syaifudin M, et al. Mutations of p53, c-kit, K-ras, and beta-catenin gene in non-Hodgkin's lymphoma of adrenal gland. Jpn J Cancer Res. 2002;93:267-74.

103. Kasaliwal R, Goroshi M, Khadilkar K, et al. Primary adrenal lymphoma: a single-center experience. Endocr Pract. 2015;21:719-24.

104. Cavanna L, Civardi G, Vallisa D, et al. Primary adrenal non-Hodgkin's lymphoma associated with autoimmune hemolytic anemia: a case diagnosed by ultrasound-guided fine needle biopsy. Ann Ital Med Int. 1999;14:298-301.

105. Kim KM, Yoon DH, Lee SG, et al. A case of primary adrenal diffuse large B-cell lymphoma achieving complete remission with rituximab-CHOP chemotherapy. J Korean Med Sci. 2009;24:525-8.

106. Cistaro A, Niccoli Asabella A, Coppolino P, et al. Diagnostic and prognostic value of 18F-FDG PET/CT in comparison with

morphological imaging in primary adrenal gland malignancies - a multicenter experience. Hell J Nucl Med. 2015;18:97-102.

107. Mansmann G, Lau J, Balk E, et al. The clinically inapparent adrenal mass: update in diagnosis and management. Endocr Rev. 2004;25:309-40.

108. Grigg AP, Connors JM. Primary adrenal lymphoma. Clin Lymphoma. 2003;4:154-60.

109. Kim YR, Kim JS, Min YH, et al. Prognostic factors in primary diffuse large B-cell lymphoma of adrenal gland treated with rituximab-CHOP chemotherapy form de consortium for improving survival of lymphoma (CISL). J Hematol Oncol. 2012;13:49.

110. Kumar R, Xiu Y, Mavi A, et al. FDG-PET imaging in primary bilateral adrenal lymphoma: a case report and review of the literature. Clin Nucl Med. 2005;30:222-30.

111. Dobrinja C, Trevisan G, Liquori G. Primary bilateral adrenal non-Hodgkin's Burkitt-like lymphoma: a rare cause of primary adrenal insufficiency. Case report and literature review. Tumori. 2007;93:625-30.

112. Kridel R, Dietrich PY. Prevention of CNS relapse in diffuse large B-cell lymphoma. Lancet Oncol. 2011;12:1258-66.

113. Boehme V, Zeynalova S, Kloess M, et al. Incidence and risk factors of central nervous system recurrence in aggressive lymphoma- a survey of 1693 patients treated in protocols of the German High-Grade Non-Hodgkin's Lymphoma Study Group (DSHNHL). Ann Oncol. 2007;18:149-57.

114. Truong B, Jolles PR, Mullaney JM. Primary adrenal lymphoma: gallium scintigraphy and correlative imaging. J Nucl Med. 1997;38:1770-1.

115. Bombardieri E, Aktolun C, Baum RP, et al. 67Ga scintigraphy: Procedure guidelines for tumour imaging. Eur J Nucl Med Mol Imaging. 2003;30:125-31.

116. Suga K, Ishikawa Y, Matsunaga N, et al. Ga-67 and I-131 adosterol scintigraphic findings of bilateral primary adrenal lymphoma. Clin Nucl Med. 2000;25:20.

117. Cheson BD, Fisher RI, Barrington SF, et al. Recommendations for initial evaluation, staging, and response assessment of Hodgkin and non-Hodgkin lymphoma: the Lugano classification. J Clin Oncol. 2014;32:3059-68.

118. Zanoni L, Cerci JJ, Fanti S. Use of PET/CT to evaluate response to therapy in lymphoma. Q J Nucl Med Mol Imaging. 2011;55:633-47.

119. Kostakoglu L, Cheson BD. State-of-the-Art Research on "Lymphomas: Role of Molecular Imaging for Staging, Prognostic Evaluation, and Treatment Response". Front Oncol. 2013;3:212.

120. Wang X. PET/CT: appropriate application in lymphoma. Chin Clin Oncol. 2015:4:4.

121. Ozimek A, Diebold J, Linke R, et al. Bilateral primary adrenal non-Hodgkin's lymphoma and primary adrenocortical carcinoma--review of the literatura preoperative differentiation of adrenal tumors. Endocr J. 2008;55:625-38.

122. Aydın K, Okutur K, Bozkurt M, et al. Primary adrenal lymphoma with secondary central nervous system involvement: a case report and review of the literature. Turk J Haematol. 2013;30:405-8.

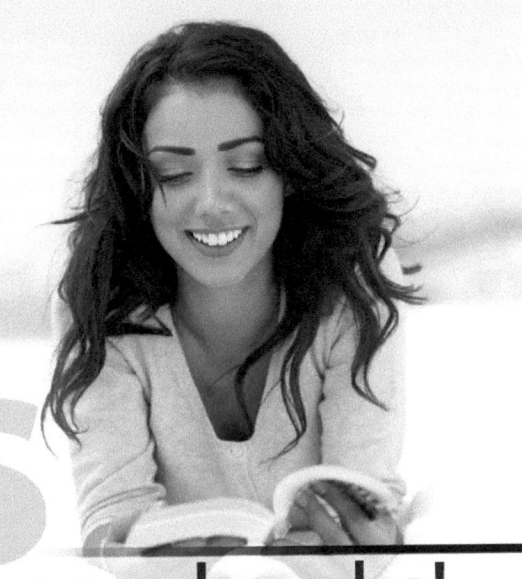
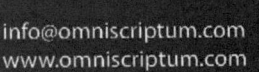 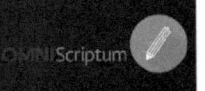

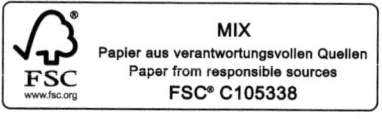